More Praise for *My Heart Is Not Asleep*

What a blessing this book is: poems earned from the threshold of love and loss, attuned to music, drenched in gorgeous imagery, and with the steady cadence of a voice willing to stay with pain and revelation. The offering of these poems, which is a true kind of gift and medicine, is one born of a courage, to return to a heart that is not asleep, that is again and again awake and open to the ravishing heartbreak of the slow loss of a beloved, and to the persistent beauty of fog and the Salish sea, of the scrape of seal whiskers on the bottom of a kayak, of huckleberry and cedar fronds and ferns, where "bright silent, urgent light rushes to touch it all." Thomas reminds us that grief and beauty are inexorable, and that patient attunement and intimacy with beauty is a path that can carry us through.
  —Anne Haven McDonnell, author of *Breath on a Coal*

Thomas Thomas's tender poems of love and grief are beautiful and powerful, sometimes overwhelming the reader with their unabashed emotion: "I know, I know, I know everything loved is to be lost / and scattered; and yet the daily lesson drums / in the blood beneath my skin." Thomas's well-crafted poems lament the shortness of life while celebrating memory's power to keep the past alive.
  —Michael Simms, author of *Strange Meadowlark*

What a poignant pleasure it is to read *My Heart Is Not Asleep,* bittersweet as many of Thomas's subjects are. I felt like I was kayaking with the poet, walking the beach with him, taking in all the natural wonders that offer him consolation on a daily basis. Thomas has captured the anguish of ambiguous loss— the endless ebbing that is dementia—but he has also captured the intimate connection that is still there for so long; and that love that never ends.
  —Ann Hedreen, author of *Her Beautiful Brain*

MY HEART IS
NOT ASLEEP

MY HEART IS
NOT ASLEEP

Thomas A. Thomas

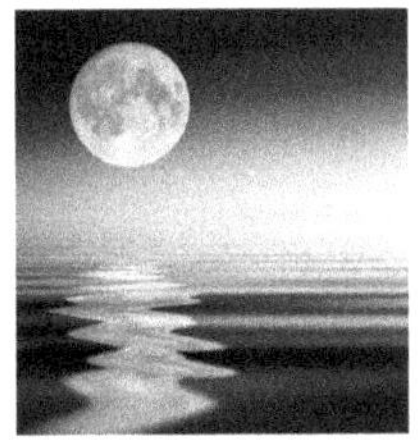

MoonPath Press

Poetry
ISBN 979-8-9899487-0-3

Cover photo: Thomas A. Thomas

Author photos: Thomas A. Thomas

Book design: Tonya Namura, using
Garamond Premier Pro (text) and Hypatia Sans Pro (display).

.

MoonPath Press, an imprint of Concrete Wolf Poetry Series, is dedicated to publishing the finest poets living in the U.S. Pacific Northwest.

MoonPath Press
c/o Concrete Wolf
PO Box 2220
Newport, OR 97365-0163

MoonPathPress@gmail.com

http://MoonPathPress.com

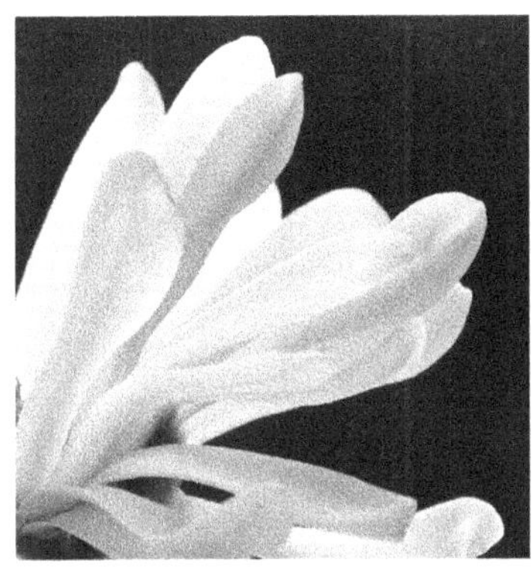

Dedicated to beloved Shaun,
for the countless memories and losses
that left the world along with her beautiful brain,
for the gift of her spirit,
and for how that light never lost its luster.

Table of Contents

MY HEART IS
NOT ASLEEP

Heart-stirred

The moment

when you glance at a woman
and she looks toward you,
and she doesn't turn away;
a slight smile moves her lips,
and because she speaks,
you have time to notice
her hair is the gold of the dry grass meadows
on mountains glimpsed through ocean mist,
and her blue-gray eyes are the color
of the Pacific, where sky and fog
melt together at the horizon;

and you say something like
I'm lost,
and she points,
takes a few steps with you,
looks in your eyes, just long enough
to remind you that your life might be,
could have been,
may yet
change in an instant,
that this tide you feel
might possibly carry you
to an ocean you may otherwise
never know.

Around Us

A beam of full moonlight falls through the skylight and
graces our pillows, our faces, lights up
dust motes, like stars turning silently above our bed.

Reflected silver lights the high knotty pine ceiling
and the knotty pine walls, each knot
you said, a galaxy.

Around us lie our halos of moonlight,
around us drift the dusty stars,
around us turn the galaxies. Outside

as it is inside our beloved bodies,
light stirs the sacred matter, the atoms germinated,
scattered by eons exploded and long gone dark stars.

Love Awakening

I wake warm & tangled with you
under our tousled covers,
come aware
of your breathing, like
slow waves sinking into sand,
over and over.

I open my eyes to the pre-dawn
wonder of you,
then close them, listening
to my own breathing
entwining
with yours.

From outside our window, a third sighing
curls into my ears.
There is now, here,

your small breath,
my small breath,

and the great breath.

Copalis Prayers

I'm walking at night,
when a breeze sets
grass blades in motion,
writing silent prayers
in the sand;

sparrows,
mice,
and insects have left
signs of their
pilgrim paths
among the burdocks.

The pearled prayer shawls
of the spiders are hung
everywhere
around the marsh
by moonlight,

and we mingle our
footprints,
mine and yours,
in dune grass
along the sand path
beside the marsh,
a prayer written by our feet,

but, come the slanted sunlight
of morning,
I find only
my own.

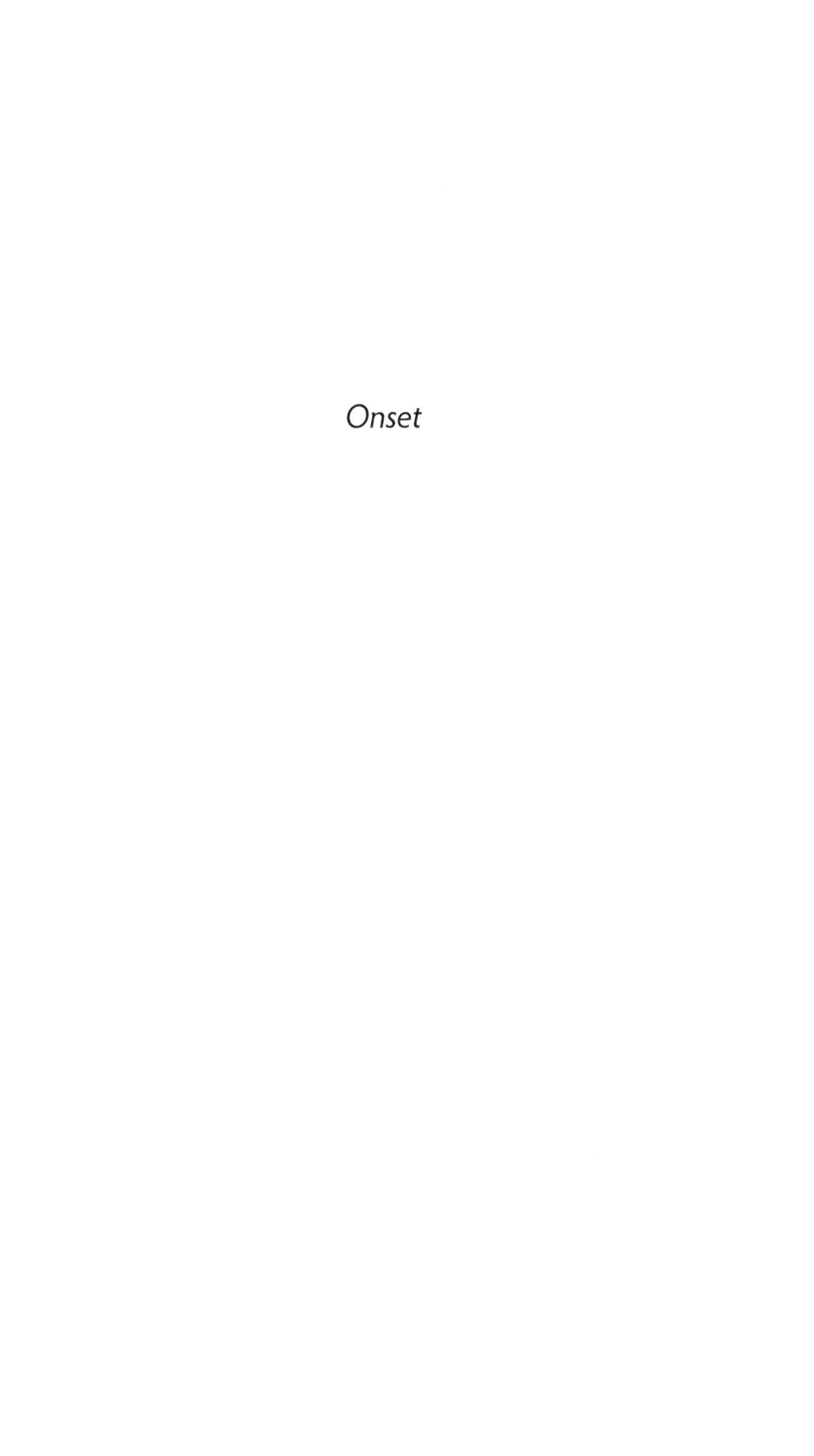

Onset

Because the Words

Because the words turn to broken glass on my tongue
and make of my voice a rusty hinge,
I write them here.

Dread darkness grows behind beloved blue eyes, under her
temple bones, beneath a forehead I still kiss, where my
nostrils seek warmth and remembered solace.

I know, I know, I know everything loved is to be lost
and scattered; and yet the daily lesson drums
in the blood beneath my skin, repeats
knots of sorrow down my bowel.

My beloved disappears, day upon night, untethered in time,
leaving language behind. And yes, because
her words are being lost,
I write these, here.

Dear Listener

This may be a story one day, but for now it's a poem,
about my beloved Shaun and her most sacred place,

and how her true father was a Dutch sailor who died
his alcoholic death on a park bench in Seattle, though

she would not be told of it for many years, so all she
knew was that he was gone, and no one spoke of him.

Her stepfather was a stupid drunk, that first word
being his more defining characteristic. Her mother

was not really a mother, for she was more interested
in being beautiful and the life of all the parties.

So Shaun was often left alone, without food or proper
clothing, or medical care, and this was even before

she had to mother her half-sister and two half-brothers
as they came along after her, one following the other.

When she was alone and hungry, which was often, she
would go to the nearby forest, and that is where

she met the spirit of a long-gone Indian chief, who was
still the guardian of the sacred woods. He watched over

her, as he did the trees and the creek called Innis, which
Shaun had to cross to reach her secret, magic temple.

Most people would not see it. They would see a big old
cedar stump in a little clearing, where sometimes the sun

would beam through the canopy to light up a huckleberry
bush that grew atop the old stump, red berries like rubies.

That is the only place where Shaun could be safe, and
eat the berries she gathered, and listen to the trees and the

creek, and the sacred stories the old chief and caretaker
of the forest would tell her on and on, over and over,

until she was fed, and she knew she was safe, and she
could sleep without fear, as the sun moved in the canopy.

Now you know where her heart grew so big, and her spirit
became unbreakable, all in this place she was not alone.

There are very few who have heard this story, and fewer
still who understand it, or imagine they think they do.

But I am sure you are one who will feel it in your heart,
and know why I cry to tell it, and what a great gift it is.

The Sirens, Before Dawn

No, my heart is not asleep.
It is awake, wide awake.
Not asleep, not dreaming—
                        —Antonio Machado

i

Some black hour past midnight and I
am dreaming at the rim of the vast silence
of Odysseus hearing those first fatal notes
in a strange distance beyond his sight

when a sound enters slowly winding
from some great darkness into my ear,
base of my skull, down my spine, pierces
my chest like an icy blade aching

something like a terrified moan, a whimper,
a keening, a ghostly ululation, wrung from
the straining throat of my love, my wife
from some deep and ancient abyss.

I gasp awake, hairs risen on my neck,
adrenaline racing my heart as the sound
echoes, reverberations fading as I reach
across to gather her head on my shoulder,

Everything is all right my love, you
are safe; you are warm and good; I am
here and I am not going anywhere
without you, dear sweetly beloved.

ii

Your forehead against my throat, your
breathing the only measure I know of time,
we sink in the warm dark, where once so
long ago I might have turned my lips to

just touch the tiny hairs of your forehead,
trace their way to your temple hollow, my
breath warming the scent of your skin,
your hair, the space behind your earlobe,

as you, still under the blanket of sleep, turn
ever so subtly toward me, arching and offering
throat, collarbone, the valley between the
breathing arcs of your breasts,

your nipples stiffening between my lips
as tongue tip traces tightened aureoles, yes
and yes, our yesses growing and burning...
in that other life we had, that gone cosmos.

My Wife's Last O

This was in the days when she
was slender as ever from anxiety
and we knew only that she was being
struck hard by something dark,

while she struggled to make plans,
make appointments, find her way
from here to there, twisted the streaks
of copper and gold still in her hair:

after lunch and before supper,
light of a golden afternoon begins
to slant inside west windows
of our house after children, music

old & soft plays under the cathedral
ceiling beneath which rests our well
used couch, my wife sitting at one
end of it, my body stretched across,

head nestled in her lap, forgetting
forgetfulness, ovarian cysts, her
atrophy, as she massages scalp and
temple, brushes hair from my forehead

rocks me warm and mesmerized,
presses my skull against her mound
and pelvic bone and her hips rise just
so gently as she closes her eyes and

Oh, she says, she says, *yes*, whispers
Ohhhh...

Evidence for the Soul in Alzheimer's Patients

> *After five years of missed diagnoses and ruling out*
> *malingering and delusion and temporary this and that,*
> *the second cranial MRI generally unremarkable until:*
> *Prominent diffuse symmetrical supratentorial cerebral*
> *atrophy involving all lobes and deep white matter*
> *in bilateral frontal lobes, abnormal for patient's age.*

She'd mostly forgotten about crying,
about her dissertation, about cooking
& teaching college and making love
& driving to meetings & appointments
& how to be with babies & children.
Then a lily might catch her eye & a smile

grow from lips to whole face & a laughing
joy burst out & finally such a radiance!
Until clouds close again; light dims,
becomes infrequent; she burns the soup,
fears neighbors on the sidewalk, thinks
I stole my car from gangsters who want

to cut my head off & leave it in our bed.
The dental hygienist asks, *how long have you two*
been married, says she sees the light between us,
the way she beams at you says she still knows you
and I hope I still look at my husband that way
when he and I have been together so many years.

Predawn, I clean up her incontinence, put on a new
brief, help her sit up at the edge of our bed, give her
her fiber gummies & brain vitamins & a Tums
for her tummy, slices of banana, nutrition shake
through a straw for my sweet baby & somehow:
when everything seems gone, there is still something.

Things come & go, mostly go, long tunnels,
dark time punctuated by bright openings
when music bursts through: a smile, a sway,
joy tears, walking the driveway on a spring
day in January, sadness tears rolling down
when we awake before dawn: *am here, here, here.*

Echolocation

My beloved says, *Please
don't do that. Oh that's not
right. She's a nice person,*
wandering endlessly.

*Okay, thank you; that is bad.
Today, today, a nice person. I'm
sorry the little baby…Do Not
go down there; that's bad…
Be nice, slowly, slowly.
We got a weirdo here: how
come? How come? Some of
the people, why? It hurts
when you talk like that:
why are you talking bad?
Right over here;*

Honey, I say, I am going to go
outside, to breathe some fresh
air, take some pictures. Do you
want to come with? *Uh huh…
Sorry. Don't do that… yep thank
you I appreciate that but I want
to go home to my home.*

So I place my camera strap
around my neck, step out on the
concrete porch, escaping down
the gravel driveway: fifty feet
to street, fifty more to bluff above
still, saltwater cove:

tide just turned to ebbing, one seal hunting,
anchovies scattering on the surface; crashing
kingfisher catching and blue heron spearing fish;
crows and woodpeckers calling; the moon just
peeking through high clouds, a grace of sunlight
on the wall of still green trees across the water;
and me wanting only to slip underwater, follow
Seal Woman down and down to her dark peace.

But I walk back, open the storm door:
*I want to go home; and it hurts, it
hurts. Oh, oh I need to go home; she's a
nice person—wonderful person—and
happy, happy; have to have it. Where is
Thomas? I surely love you, I surely do
love if you don't mind, if I say hi. Hi
honey bunny, I want to go home.*

The Years

In a Time

There are times when I feel trapped in time.
And this is one of those times, the year 2020,
a time in the impossible future I expected not
to be alive to see, and the month is August
and August is the month and time of litany.

It is the month of my one wedding, the month
of gaining a son who could have been thirty-one.
It is the month of our first walk along the salt
shore together, and of my beloved's first illness,
harbinger of worse to come, month of our lost

mortgage, of bankruptcy, August of learning
my only brother had renal cell carcinoma, would
follow my father to that hard darkness so soon,
the month of disability determination, August
of a diagnosis at last, terribly final as it is.

And it is still the month berries ripen along
humid vines, corn ears swell in steamy fields,
as fawns fatten out of their spots, gorging on
clover blossoms and dandelion blooms, as seal
pups bask between fishing lessons, as fingerlings

flash to avoid shadows, as kingfisher young
learn not to make shadows as they dive, it is
the month apples begin to blush at the thought
of falling, time of joy upon joy, joy upon sorrow,
time of sorrow, time of love upon love upon love.

What Remains

After so many losses,
nights like burnt wicks,
days too, I cajole her out
on a sunny late morning.

These she notices:
wild cherry petals falling like snow
in cedar shadows, drifting onto
sword ferns, and columbine

jewels from last night's rain
beaded and gleaming there
on the velvet underside
of a madrona leaf,

the forget-me-nots blue,
and some pink, standing around
the pole at the end of the drive
where I didn't mow,

the scent from the daphne
bush in bloom, a tiny pinch
I hold below her nostrils, *yes
beautiful,* she says.

Inside again, simple sharing,
me spooning vanilla ice cream
drizzled with chocolate syrup
for her, her tears of joy.

The Right Word

The right word is not *shroud*...
not today at least, and not
cocoon, though the cloth is
wound round the body on
the hospital bed. No, the word
is only *sheet*, right for this
first day of a separate bed,

in the guest room at the other
end of our rented home.

The right word is not *rain*,
though the radar says so, not
this afternoon, when imagined
droplets touch skin, as I mow
late grass, dandelions, not
drizzle nor *mist*, but *virga*,
rain that falls yet does not.

Good morning, my Love

(You try to say this as if
it were not the last time)

Here's your glasses, as you slip
them onto her nose (again, as if)

Then you have her sitting (yes)
on the edge of the bed,

(knowing) and brush her hair
long & slowly back of her shoulders.

And when her eyes close, you
touch her lips with a strawberry.

(which is, this one and only moment,
all and everything we know)

I will always want one more kiss

I say this to my wife as my lips leave hers,
as I prepare to leave her in her care home bed,
and it must be true, say the tears on my cheeks.

And then I kiss again, and tell her yes, *it's true,*
despite her closed eyes and open—though
speechless—lips, I do so always want one more.

It is also a kiss when I turn at the door to
look back, at the body restless, twitching, her
breath sometimes hissing between lips, lost teeth.

And when I open the front door, a gust of spring
—raindrops and spinning plum petals—is yes,
another kiss, for which yes, I give thanks.

My bare feet on young grass and sun-warm soil,
a walk back home is kisses for the earth, as
daffodils and camellia are kisses for my eyes,

eyes that are shedding brine tears again, or still,
as truly they catch the pollen wafting in kind
breezes, from fir and maple and cherry trees.

And to stand beside a flower bed memory of my
beloved is a kiss, and a longing which is still
and again, another desire for, yes, one more kiss.

Knowing sleep will not come again

though the windows of my bedroom
remain black and blank, I draw my
body from the warmth where you are

not, still not, always not,
and leave the lights off, let my fingers
find yesterday's clothes at the foot

of the vast vacant bed: socks, jeans,
tee-shirt, sweater, and slip on
the shoes next to the nightstand then

feel my way along to the kitchen table
where just enough sky light falls
to reveal the charcoal jacket hung dry

on the back of a bentwood chair, and
push my arms into it and open the door
to the breath of just barely twilight fog,

tiny droplets touching so lightly as
to feel almost imaginary, as I close
the kitchen door behind, and step

into the silence of calm wind, fog.
A couple scuffs of steps whisper on
concrete before the crunch of gravel

underfoot, before the soft path under
fir trees, where fog drops land, tick
and tap upon late winter maple leaves.

Through the white noise of the dark
fog, barred owl says *good night night,*
as raven chuckles his good matins

to anyone beneath the reticent cedars,
cormorants grunt awake across the cove.
The steps to invisible water are empty

as our bed afloat in the cabin drifting
beneath our oak up the stone gray hill,
as unseen, a heron complains and goes,

startles my heart—which whispers
once again, *I was looking for you.*

When I Left Her There

It seemed over, and
I thought I should
fly straight up in
pure shirtless joy
along the foamy
lace of summer's
beach as waves
danced ashore, me
leaping & dancing
on frothing light,
but a silence comes.

And grief like a shriek,
like a rush of feathers,
like talons sinking
through my skin to
bone and muscle,
strikes me to stillness
to stare at those same
surges of ocean light,
past which I might
swim out to darkness.

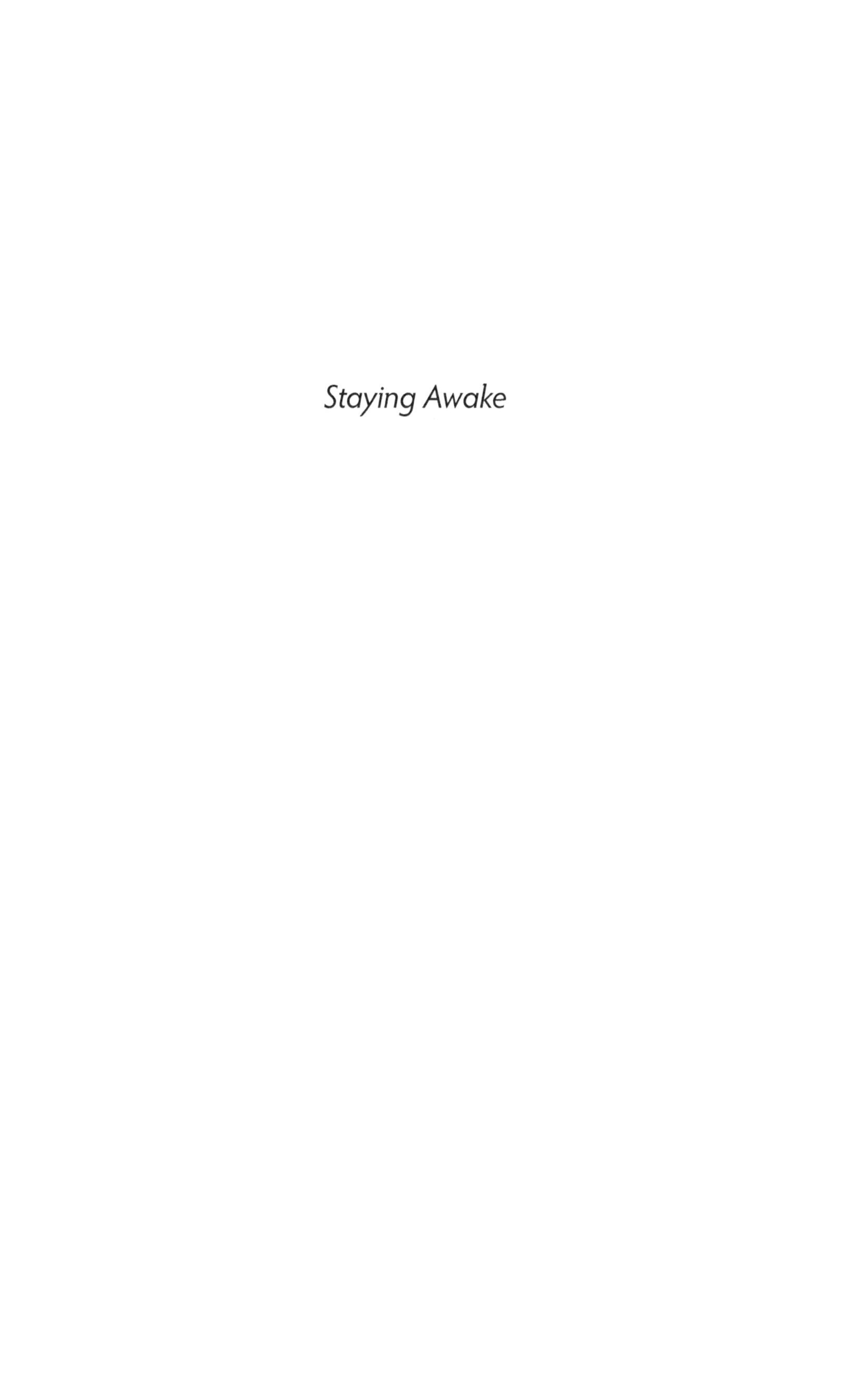

Staying Awake

Instead of god

say heron, say kingfisher,
say that was the tenth summer
my wife was dying and I
was not.

Instead of god say
a name, like Ann or Grace
or Joy, say the one who broke
me open in a new way this
wholly unexpected time.

Instead of god say love
let joy in the side door and she
sits in the kitchen now in the
warmth of fresh bread and
cinnamon and honey.

Instead of god say only
desire, want, say pomegranate,
poplar tree, say stay, say please,
say thank you, say love again
dark and light and forever.

Communion

She can't talk anymore
not a word,

has not said
my name in years,

not in words, anyway,
but her wrinkled

forehead and knitted
eyebrows know my thumb

and I hope she knows my
voice, as I break to bits

soft chocolate to
place on her tongue,

bringing perhaps
a smile I almost see,

perhaps a sigh
I can almost hear.

Restacking the Wood

I slept through something in the night
that spilled split cedar and alder
onto the grass, a whole row tumbled.

Fears and plans and strategies and
mitigations demand my waking: yet
there's nothing to be done, even futile.

So stacking wood is something: in jeans,
boots, work shirt, and gloves, out back
in chilly morning air, I begin.

My Returning

after Laura Tohe

I have been in this other story for a very long time, a story
mostly written by others mostly because I let them...though
that does not mean the story lacked meaning or lacked
sweetness or bitterness or even deep love. Wait. Listen.

I only mean that it is passing into the past, even the future
is passing away. The people of that story have gone, are
going, whether they have walked away or been scattered
in the cornfields along the river, or in the river itself, or
on the mountain snows, or the winds of dry canyons. I am

returning to this place someone calls now and some other
calls the body and maybe it is these and something else
too: a flower at the highest blossoming in the moment she
turns toward death. I am, I am, I am not separate, I am
not apart. I am joining, not dividing. I am sitting in an oak
tree watching, on the river floating from forest to sea, I am

flat on the ocean sand. I am beach, motion of water, motion
of stars, motion of pelican, fish, seal, snail, beetle, butterfly.
I am so welcome, I am invisible.

Picking Joy

It begins with a huckleberry like a ruby,
red gleam in green beneath dark fir
canopy where even August heat cannot
reach, and leads my eye to another

jewel and another and another light
in a clearing where a sunbeam makes
leaves incandesce upon nurse stump
altar, shadowed temple where she prayed,

and I listen to a new silence until barely
a puff of wind at first lifts my hair, then
growing, lifts cedar boughs, stirs ferns,
brings down leaves from alder and maple

that tumble brown and yellow down onto
the bare earth path now visible, winding
toward a tawny clearing beneath wind-
stirred branches and dancing fern fronds

I wade through to reach the bright meadow
ringed with blackberry runners and vines
tangled and dense reaching up through
alder and cedar, as spider silk streamers

gleaming dazzle my eyes and a sweet scent
tickles my nostrils as dark berries shine
among green leaves and purple vines, and
I lean forward to reach between thorns,

touch a berry, tap, grasp between fingers
and thumb, squeeze to test, tug so lightly
so as not to burst juice from drupelets
and this one holds on, doesn't drop so I

let it stay to ripen for another being who
may even now be recalling this vine encircled
meadow where, as it happens at this moment,
I remember my berry pilgrim wife from before

the sweet lobes of her brain withered and
neuron vines tangled like these dying as they
climb upward, and I am pierced knowing
one cannot pluck this joy without that grief.

Something Turns

Something turns in the cells of ferns
and birds and blackberries
under the burnt orange sky.

Smoky air erases the idea of horizon
where I've walked to the liminal
zone of beige grass and green woods.

Thorny vines have climbed among
hawthorn trees and alder saplings
and the purple fruit rests there.

I am not so much picking berries
as touching to find those that
give themselves to my cupped palm.

It seems I have always been doing
this for my dearly beloved, finding
sweetness at the edge of somewhere.

Air hot and smoky from distant fires:
sun orange high in the sky, not
dream, not nightmare, incarnation.

Kayak Reverie

The sun is not yet high
but the cirrus are,

as I slice Salish salt water,
pull a paddle to push my

kayak into wind and
rising tide, as sunlight

flows upon my skin,
silvers fish in mid-air

where an osprey wheels
around sundogs and crows

and seagull calls mingle
with whistles and caws,

the sound of an oyster barge
thrumming under all this,

when a seal woman whispers
her whiskers along my hull,

splashes her somersault
tail to send water sparks

up and up, gold drops falling
through blue air to sudden

silence. Wind stops riffling
water to let it be mirror of

cirrus sky, as crows leave
off chasing the sailing away

long winged osprey, and the
barge stops rumbling and

my paddle, and everything
stops, a moment, two, then

even my breathing, here
between sea world, its

dark electricity flowing
beneath sky world, where

bright silent, urgent light
rushes to touch it all.

Storm Song (just now)

Driving home in sunshine, thunderhead
bears toward the highway and me, wind
drops flashes of dazzle on my windshield.

And all I hear is music and you, saxophone
lips that tickle your earlobe, double bass
fingers make soft percussions on your spine,

flute breaths ripple in your throat, and sighs
lead guitar notes to float down waist & hips
along my thighs sustained on yours, then

drum rumble...electric reverberation of skin,
a rain hiss of brush on snare, and we are
song and I am skyward singing you.

Last of the Kayak Soliloquies

Months have spun past, silence
clear and cold and resonant
like air after the bell
is no longer heard.

So many blessings to count today,
adrift on a mirror of salt water,
so much good I must
remember to remember.

And sometimes it takes such
a day as this to help do so,
a day both glorious
and still.

My paddling waves and those of
the geese with their watchful eyes
are the largest out here.
One small plane flew over.

I heard a family walking along
the gravel shore, parents pointing
the birds out to the children.
And now there's almost

nothing to hear. This moment
it's me, and feathers on ripples,
and the last fog burning off
like thoughts of her.

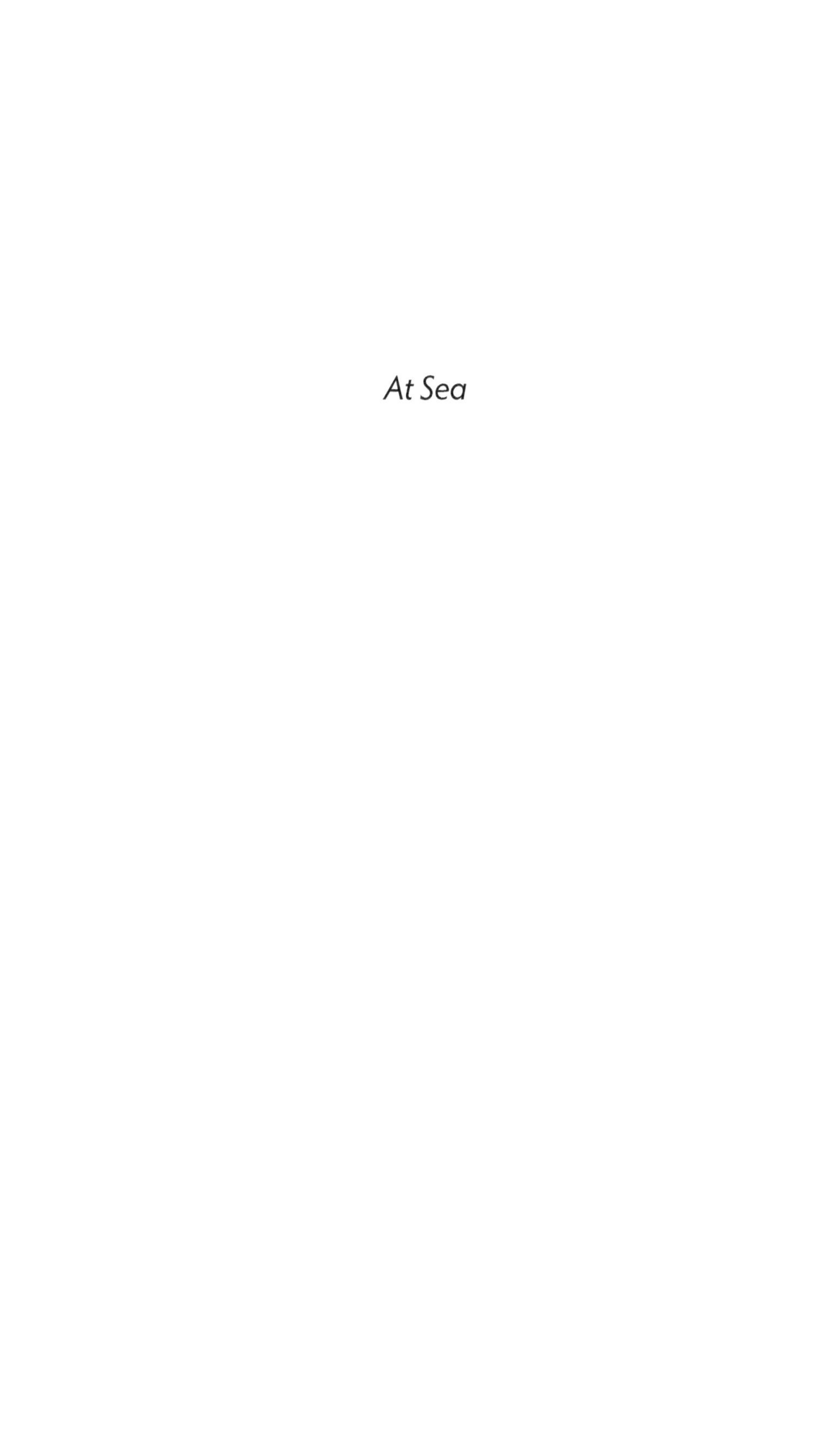

At Sea

Dream Under Venus

We've had a reflective dinner
at sunset, at a glass table
outside the restaurant
together as the sun went
down among the masts
in the still harbor. The waiter
has come and gone.

I stand and with fingertips
brush bangs back from
your forehead. You stand
and take my hand. We take
a few steps together along
the old boardwalk. We smile
and look at one another

in the almost darkness,
and then our hands fall
to our sides as they let go
of each other. As we turn
and walk toward our
separate cars in the now dark,
a wind or wave moves boats,

sets the riggings to tapping
on the aluminum of the masts:
little bells.

Death's Questions

Can you hold her now deformed feet
with the same reverence you cupped
her breasts in longing?

Will you still kiss those affectless lips
as fervently as when they were warm
and kissed you back?

Remembering the restored turquoise
earrings you hung on her lobes, do
you touch her ears devotedly still?

As she leaves you with my shadow,
are you able to smooth the sheets
as always you did, in love?

Tides

She opens her
blue-green eyes
and I feel the sea
tug at my ribs,
though
she remains
in the little boat
of her hospital bed.

Gratitude

With admiration and thankfulness for the providers, poets,
and seers who kept me upright:

Dr. James Ingersoll, who helps me still, with weaving a tale
in the tapestry of my life. To Laura Vaillancourt, navigator
extraordinaire of our eldercare journey. Ann Hedreen, whose
book *Her Beautiful Brain* helped light my path.

Also with huge gratefulness to the Live Like a Poet critique
and encouragement group, founded by Joanne M. Clarkson,
with members Patrick Dixon, Carol R. Sunde, Wesley Jones,
and Bridgit Lacy.

Great thanks to Dr. Devika Brendon for her support and
guidance in the formative days of this collection. Thanks
to Anne Haven McDonnell in the later days, with Poets
on the River. And I cannot overstate my thanks for the
encouragement of Rena Priest, at Fishtrap Summer 2023, and
for Sean Hill, at Elk River Writers Workshop, August 2023.

Profound thanks to Claudia Putnam for enthusiastic, expert,
and energetic assistance in crafting the final shape of the
manuscript.

Love also to the caregivers who came into Shaun's and my
life when needed, often despite their own woundedness and
trauma, who gave me hope of survival through the darkest
days and nights.

Acknowledgements

The author gratefully acknowledges the following publications where poems from this collection first appeared:

The Banyan Review, Issue 5: Spring 2021: "Instead of god"

FemAsiaMagazine.com, October 25, 2020: "In a time"

Gyroscope Review, Summer 2022: "Kayak Reverie"

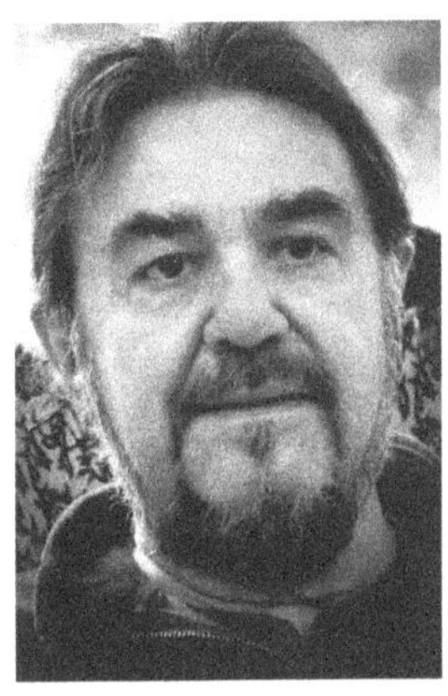

About the Author

Thomas A. Thomas, born in Illinois to a medical doctor mother and a ballet dancer father, spent a lot of time off by himself in the woods, prairies, and fields, day and night, in all seasons.

Thomas found his way to the University of Michigan, where he studied with Donald Hall, and Gregory Orr, and workshopped some poems with Robert Bly. He won Minor and Major Hopwood Awards in Poetry, and his poem "Approaching Here" was choreographed and performed at UM.

After a couple of years of madness in New York City, he found his way to the Pacific Northwest, where he has made his home for over 40 years. He is now delighted to be a Board Member for the Olympia Poetry Network, and to be active in numerous online poetry and photography groups.

His works appear in print and online, including video recordings, most recently in *Gyroscope Review, Blue Heron Review, Cirque Journal, Vox Populi, TheBanyanReview.org*, and *FemAsiaMagazine.com*, as well as anthologies in English and in translation to Spanish, Serbian, and Bengali. He has been nominated for both Best of the Net and The Pushcart Prize.

This collection of poems regards his experience of caring
for his wife for over a decade, up to the present time, as she
gradually succumbs to extreme early onset Alzheimer's disease.

Visit Thomas online at https://linktr.ee/thomasathomas

www.ingramcontent.com/pod-product-compliance
Lightning Source LLC
Chambersburg PA
CBHW041651150726
48005CB00013BA/1618